NAVIGATING VULVAR CANCER WITH CONFIDENCE AND CARE

Empowering Insights And Strategies For Confronting Cancer Health Challenges For Female Genitals Recovery

DR. WESLEY IAN

© [2024] [Wesley Ian].

All rights reserved. Without the publisher's prior written consent, no portion of this publication may be copied, distributed, or transmitted in any way, including by photocopying, recording, or other mechanical or electronic means, with the exception of brief quotations used in critical reviews and other noncommercial uses allowed by copyright law. To request permission, please send an email to [your contact information].

DISCLAIMER

The information in this book is not meant to replace professional medical advice, diagnosis, or treatment; rather, it is meant mainly for general informational reasons. If you have any questions about a medical problem, you should always consult your doctor or another trained health expert. Don't ever discount expert medical advice or put off getting it because of something you've read in this book.

Any negative effects or repercussions arising from the usage of the material provided herein are not the responsibility of the book's author or publisher. It should be noted by readers that the material in this book is not all-inclusive and might not address every facet of the subject. Furthermore, new research may have an impact on how health concerns are understood or treated because medical knowledge is always changing.

No particular test, treatment, method, or product mentioned in this book is endorsed or promoted by the author or publisher. The reader assumes all risk associated with using the information included in this book.

Before making any big decisions regarding your health, it's crucial to speak with a licensed healthcare provider. The relationship between a patient and their healthcare practitioner should not be replaced by this book, nor is it meant to offer medical advice.

The opinions presented in this book are the author's and may not necessarily represent those of the publisher. Any errors, omissions, or inaccuracies in the information in this book are not the responsibility of the author or publisher.

It is recommended that readers independently confirm any information contained in this book and speak with a healthcare provider about their specific medical needs and state of health.

TABLE OF CONTENTS

CHAPTER ONE 12

  INTRODUCTION TO VULVAR CANCER 12

    COMPREHENDING VULVAR CANCER.............................12

    TYPES AND DEFINITIONS OF VULVAR CANCER................13

    REASONS AND DANGER FACTORS................................14

    SYMPTOMS AND INDICATIONS 14

CHAPTER TWO 16

  THE VULVAR CANCER DIAGNOSIS 16

    IDENTIFYING AND FILTERING 16

    DIAGNOSTIC TECHNIQUES AND EXAMINATIONS..............17

    ANALYZING TEST FINDINGS..18

CHAPTER THREE 20

  GETTING AROUND THE MEDICAL TRIP..............................20

    ASSEMBLING YOUR MEDICAL STAFF 20

    OVERVIEW OF TREATMENT OPTIONS 21

    MAKING KNOWLEDGEABLE CHOICES 22

CHAPTER FOUR 24

  ASPECTS OF EMOTION AND PSYCHOLOGY 24

    MANAGING A DIAGNOSIS OF VULVAR CANCER................24

    SPEAKING WITH CLOSE RELATIVES 25

    REQUESTING EMOTIONAL ASSISTANCE 27

CHAPTER FIVE...28

  METHODS OF TREATMENT...28

    SURGERY 28

RADIATION TREATMENT 29

CHEMOTHERAPY AND ADDITIONAL DRUGS 30

CHAPTER SIX...32

HAVING VULVAR CANCER AND GETTING BY.................................32

CONTROLLING ADVERSE REACTIONS 32

SUSTAINING LIFE QUALITY 33

COMBINING COMPLEMENTARY MEDICINE 34

CHAPTER SEVEN 36

INTIMACY AND SEXUALITY 36

HANDLING MODIFICATIONS IN SEXUAL FUNCTION 36

SPEAKING WITH PARTNERS..37

REGAINING CLOSENESS...38

CHAPTER EIGHT 40

DIETARY ADVICE..40

DURING TREATMENT, NUTRITION 40

PARTICULAR ATTENTION FOR PATIENTS WITH VULVAR CANCER......41

MEAL PLANS AND RECIPES..42

CHAPTER NINE 44

USEFUL ADVICE FOR EVERYDAY LIFE.................................44

HANDLING EVERYDAY DIFFICULTIES 44

KEEPING YOUR INDEPENDENCE 45

MANAGING TREATMENT AND WORK 46

CHAPTER TEN 48

RESILIENCE AND CONTINUED CARE 48

AFTER TREATMENT LIFE 48

FREQUENT INSPECTIONS AND SURVEILLANCE 49

PROLONGED SURVIVAL 50

ABOUT THE BOOK

The thorough manual "Navigating Vulvar Cancer with Confidence and Care" is a priceless tool for anyone navigating the obstacles of vulvar cancer. The book, which is written with empathy and accuracy, covers a wide range of important vulvar cancer-related topics and provides patients, caregivers, and medical professionals with a framework of support in addition to a multitude of information.

The beginning of the book clearly states its goal, establishing the tone for a resource that goes beyond simple information sharing. By giving patients with vulvar cancer a road map for comprehending, negotiating, and eventually overcoming the challenges of their medical path, it seeks to empower those who are facing this disease.

The book is laid up in an approachable way, starting with an introduction to vulvar cancer. In-depth chapters on definitions, types, causes, and risk factors make sure readers understand the subtleties of the illness.

The book leads readers through the diagnostic procedure and provides them with the necessary knowledge to understand detection, screening, and test result interpretation.

The thorough examination of the medical journey, which highlights the need to assemble a healthcare team and make well-informed treatment selections, is a noteworthy aspect. Understanding the psychological and emotional toll that receiving a vulvar cancer diagnosis may have, the book dedicates to coping tactics, how to communicate with loved ones, and how to get the necessary emotional support.

Additionally, the guide offers comprehensive insights into various treatment techniques, demystifying radiation therapy, chemotherapy, and surgery. The book covers the whole health and well-being of people with vulvar cancer in addition to its clinical components. This includes managing side effects, preserving quality of life, and incorporating complementary therapies.

The delicate subject of sexuality and intimacy is given extra consideration, with helpful guidance on how to handle changes in sexual function, interact with partners, and regain intimacy.

The book also offers nutritional advice specifically designed to meet the needs of individuals with vulvar cancer, including suggestions for during treatment, things to think about and even doable recipes and meal plans.

The book's dedication to providing comprehensive help is demonstrated by the useful advice for everyday living included. These insights improve the resilience of people with vulvar cancer, from overcoming everyday obstacles to juggling jobs and treatment.

Ultimately, the book offers a survivorship and follow-up care path, looking beyond the immediate obstacles. Discussions about long-term survivorship, routine check-ups, and life after treatment offer a thorough roadmap for people navigating the challenges of life after cancer.

"Navigating Vulvar Cancer with Confidence and Care" is more than just a manual; it's a travel companion that provides information, encouragement, and a path forward for those who need it.

CHAPTER ONE

INTRODUCTION TO VULVAR CANCER

Vulvar cancer is a type of cancer that affects the external female genitalia. It is a complicated medical problem with many facets that necessitate a thorough understanding to fully navigate. The vulva, which includes the external genitalia, can develop malignancies of many kinds, each with its special difficulties in terms of diagnosis and therapy. This introduction analyzes the signs and symptoms that may suggest the presence of vulvar cancer as well as its definition, forms, and possible causes. It also discusses risk factors for the development of vulvar cancer.

COMPREHENDING VULVAR CANCER

The labia, clitoris, and vaginal opening are among the tissues of the vulva that can develop into vulvar carcinoma, an uncommon but dangerous type of cancer. The vulva is an essential component of the reproductive anatomy of women, and any anomalies or malignant growths in this area can have a significant impact on a woman's health. Examining the pathophysiology, etiology, and several contributing variables to the formation of vulvar cancer is necessary to comprehend its complexities.

TYPES AND DEFINITIONS OF VULVAR CANCER

A collection of cancerous tumors that develop in the vulvar tissues is referred to as vulvar cancer. Squamous cell carcinoma is the most common type of these tumors, and other less common varieties like adenocarcinoma, melanoma, and sarcoma are also included in this general classification. Adenocarcinoma begins in the glandular cells, whereas squamous cell carcinoma grows from the thin, flat cells lining the vulva's surface. Despite being uncommon, melanoma and sarcoma need to be treated with specific care because of their unique features.

A thorough comprehension of these kinds is necessary for precise diagnosis and individualized treatment plans.

REASONS AND DANGER FACTORS

Numerous variables, including genetic, environmental, and behavioral ones, can contribute to vulvar cancer. High-risk strains of the human papillomavirus (HPV) are persistently infectious and have been linked to vulvar cancer, especially squamous cell carcinoma. Additional risk factors include smoking, aging, immune system weakness, chronic skin disorders, and age, with an increased occurrence in older women. Deciphering how these elements interact can help develop early detection and preventative treatments.

SYMPTOMS AND INDICATIONS

For an early diagnosis and successful treatment of vulvar cancer, it is essential to recognize the symptoms and indicators of the disease. Individuals may have vulvar area pain, soreness, or persistent itching. Potential problems include changes in skin color or thickness, the appearance of lumps or lesions, and bleeding that is not related to menstruation. Given that these symptoms may coincide with benign illnesses, it is crucial to seek medical assistance for a comprehensive evaluation as soon as such changes are seen.

A comprehensive examination of the definition, kinds, causes, and symptoms of vulvar cancer is necessary to fully comprehend the disease. Through an exploration of the intricacies of this ailment, both medical experts and individuals can strive towards prompt identification, enhanced therapeutic results, and an enhanced standard of living for vulvar cancer patients.

CHAPTER TWO
THE VULVAR CANCER DIAGNOSIS
IDENTIFYING AND FILTERING

Vulvar cancer is a relatively rare form of cancer that affects the external genitalia of women. Owing to its rarity and the absence of standard screening protocols designed only for vulvar cancer, diagnosis frequently depends on patients' and healthcare professionals' awareness of symptoms. Consistent gynecological exams are essential for detecting any anomalies or modifications in the vulvar area. Medical practitioners may visually examine the vulva to look for any atypical lesions, discoloration, or other indications that might require more research.

To enable people to be watchful of changes in their bodies, self-examinations are promoted in addition to clinical examinations. It is recommended that women report any sustained itching, pain, or the appearance of lumps or sores in the vulvar area. Self-examinations can help identify anomalies early and encourage people to seek medical assistance promptly, but they should not be used in place of professional medical evaluations.

DIAGNOSTIC TECHNIQUES AND EXAMINATIONS

Healthcare professionals may suggest particular diagnostic procedures to ascertain the nature of the vulvar alterations if suspicious symptoms or anomalies are found during routine examinations or self-assessments. A biopsy is a frequent diagnostic procedure in which a small sample of tissue is taken for analysis in a lab from the affected area. Determining whether the changes seen are benign, precancerous, or suggestive of vulvar cancer is much easier with the help of the biopsy.

Another diagnostic method for evaluating vulvar abnormalities is colposcopy. In this treatment, the vulvar tissues are closely examined using a magnification device called a colposcope. If any suspicious lesions are found during a colposcopy, medical professionals may also take a biopsy.

To ascertain the extent of the malignancy, imaging techniques like positron emission tomography (PET), magnetic resonance imaging (MRI), or computed tomography (CT) scans may be used, particularly if there are signs that the disease has spread to neighboring lymph nodes or other organs.

ANALYZING TEST FINDINGS

An important part of the vulvar cancer diagnosis procedure is interpreting test results. To identify cancer cells and define the precise type and stage of the disease, pathologists examine biopsy samples. The outcomes of imaging investigations help with treatment planning and offer important information regarding the degree of tumor spread.

When vulvar cancer is identified, the stage of the illness becomes crucial in determining the best course of therapy. Evaluation of the tumor's size, extent of invasion into adjacent tissues, and presence of metastases to distant organs or lymph nodes are all part of the staging process. Oncologists can create a customized treatment plan that combines chemotherapy, radiation therapy, surgery, or a mix of these modalities with the use of the staging process.

When interpreting test results, patients and healthcare practitioners must communicate effectively. Precise elucidations of the results, available therapies, and probable consequences enable patients to make knowledgeable decisions regarding their medical care. A multimodal approach to therapy and the assistance of medical professionals guarantee that patients with vulvar cancer receive thorough and sensitive care throughout their journey.

CHAPTER THREE

GETTING AROUND THE MEDICAL TRIP

ASSEMBLING YOUR MEDICAL STAFF

Putting together a strong healthcare team is essential when starting a medical journey. This team is made up of a variety of experts who are essential to providing complete care and assistance. A primary care physician usually acts as the main point of contact and is at the center of this team. This individual manages the team's overall health, works with professionals to plan, and helps team members communicate.

Because they each provide experience in a particular medical specialty, specialists become essential members of the healthcare team. Depending on the nature of the medical journey, these specialists may include neurologists, surgeons, oncologists, or other healthcare providers. For the patient to receive comprehensive and well-coordinated care, team members must collaborate and communicate well with one another.

Including various support services in the healthcare team building process is common, in addition to medical personnel. Depending on the person's medical needs, this could involve nurses, social workers, PTs, and even dietitians. In many circumstances, patients may decide to engage friends, family, or mental health experts in their healthcare support system. Social and emotional support is also very important.

OVERVIEW OF TREATMENT OPTIONS

Having a thorough awareness of all of the treatment options available is essential for navigating the medical path. Learning about different treatment techniques, from conventional to alternative therapy, is an important first step. Depending on the type of illness, conventional therapies may involve drugs, surgery, chemotherapy, or radiation therapy.

More and more research is being done on complementary or alternative therapies as part of the overall therapeutic strategy. These could include lifestyle changes, herbal medicines, chiropractic adjustments, and acupuncture. Patients must consult with their healthcare provider about these options to make sure they are in line with current treatment plans and to prevent any conflicts or negative consequences.

Clinical trials and experimental treatments are an additional avenue of therapy consideration for individuals. Clinical trial participation can advance medical research and give access to cutting-edge therapies. To make an informed choice, one must, however, balance the dangers and potential benefits and speak with medical experts.

MAKING KNOWLEDGEABLE CHOICES

A key component of successfully navigating the medical journey is making educated decisions. To do this, patients must actively engage in their healthcare decisions and maintain current knowledge about their conditions, available treatments, and possible results. Patients and healthcare providers must have open and honest communication, and patients should feel free to voice any concerns they may have and ask for clarification when needed.

Making educated judgments requires gathering information from trustworthy sources, such as support groups, credible websites, and medical experts. By being able to comprehend their diagnosis, available treatments, and possible adverse effects, people are more equipped to actively participate in shared decision-making with their healthcare team.

In some cases, getting a second opinion can be helpful because it can offer fresh viewpoints and insights into the best course of action. Making decisions must be approached holistically, taking into account not only the medical implications but also the effects on quality of life, individual values, and long-term objectives.

Creating a solid healthcare team, being aware of your options for treatment, and making well-informed decisions all work together to create a seamless medical experience.

CHAPTER FOUR

ASPECTS OF EMOTION AND PSYCHOLOGY

MANAGING A DIAGNOSIS OF VULVAR CANCER

For some people, learning they have vulvar cancer can be an extremely taxing experience. The emotional toll is frequently complex, including feelings of worry, anxiety, and future uncertainty. Navigating through a wide range of complex emotions and attending to the practical requirements of therapy and healthcare are all part of coping with such a diagnosis. People could struggle with a sense of loss related to perceived normalcy in their lives as well as physical health.

Understanding the nature of vulvar cancer, the available treatments, and the possible consequences is often the first step in the coping process. With this knowledge, people might feel more in control of their lives and be able to make wise decisions. Coping, however, includes more than just learning about the illness; it also entails accepting the emotional cost of it. When patients deal with the changes in their lives, they may feel a variety of emotions, such as despair, remorse, and rage.

Coping mechanisms may also entail obtaining psychological assistance, such as counseling or therapy. Professionals in mental health can offer a secure environment where people can process the emotional effects of their diagnosis, express their thoughts, and create coping strategies.

Making connections with support groups made up of people who have encountered or are currently experiencing comparable difficulties can also provide a feeling of belonging and understanding.

SPEAKING WITH CLOSE RELATIVES

For the patient and their loved ones, good communication is essential upon receiving a vulvar cancer diagnosis. Such news must be disclosed with a careful combination of compassion, openness, and assurance. Family members may go through a range of emotions themselves, from astonishment and worry to wanting to offer steadfast support.

In these kinds of circumstances, communication that works must be based on honesty. To promote understanding between patients and their loved ones, patients may find it helpful to discuss their thoughts, anxieties, and treatment plans with them.

Promoting open communication makes it easier for people to express their feelings and makes it easier to create a supportive environment. Family members can also be extremely helpful in providing practical support, including going to doctor's appointments with the patient or helping with everyday tasks.

But it's important to understand that different people have different communication styles, and some people may find it difficult to verbally convey their emotions. In these situations, other forms of communication, like writing or participating in group activities, might offer a channel for connection and expression.

REQUESTING EMOTIONAL ASSISTANCE

Seeking emotional support from multiple sources is often necessary to navigate the emotional terrain following a vulvar cancer diagnosis. Guidance for managing the psychological components of the condition can be customized with professional support from psychologists, counselors, or therapists. These experts can support people in exploring and comprehending their feelings, creating coping mechanisms, and attempting to keep a positive attitude in life.

Seeking solace from friends, family, and support groups helps provide a network of emotional sustenance in addition to professional care. Making connections with people who have had comparable difficulties can provide a special kind of support, encouraging a feeling of unity and mutual understanding. It's critical to understand that asking for emotional assistance is a proactive move toward comprehensive well-being rather than a show of weakness.

CHAPTER FIVE
METHODS OF TREATMENT
SURGERY

Surgery is a widely used therapeutic approach for several medical disorders, from benign tumors to cancers that can be fatal. The choice to have surgery is frequently made in concert with the patient's medical team, taking into account various aspects like the type of ailment, its stage, and the patient's general health. Patients should anticipate having in-depth conversations with their doctors before the treatment, during which they will explore the advantages and disadvantages of the surgery as well as any possible alternatives.

Patients may require preoperative exams, such as imaging studies, blood tests, and other diagnostic assessments, to be ready for surgery. Clear instructions on pre-surgery protocols, such as fasting or stopping specific drugs, are usually given by surgeons.

Anesthesia is administered during the actual surgical procedure to guarantee the patient's comfort and security.

Depending on the intricacy of the procedure, patients can expect a range of experiences throughout the critical post-surgery recovery phase. This can entail physical therapy, pain treatment, and follow-up visits to track development and handle any possible issues. Recovery involves an emotional component as well, and support systems like groups or counseling may be suggested.

RADIATION TREATMENT

High radiation doses are used in radiation therapy, a therapeutic method, to target and destroy aberrant cells. This method is frequently used in cancer treatment, either on its own or in conjunction with other therapies like chemotherapy or surgery. Radiation therapy's basic idea is to harm the targeted cells' DNA, which stops them from proliferating and eventually causes their demise.

Patients usually go through a thorough planning phase before starting radiation therapy, where doctors accurately identify the target area and create a personalized treatment plan. Although treatment sessions are often brief—just a few minutes long—the whole time may take several weeks. Side effects that patients may encounter include nausea, exhaustion, and skin changes; they are closely watched over and handled by the medical staff.

The efficacy of radiation therapy is attributed to its capacity to target cancer cells specifically while causing the least amount of damage to nearby healthy tissues. Technological developments like intensity-modulated radiation therapy (IMRT) and proton therapy have improved patient outcomes and quality of life by improving precision and lowering adverse effects.

CHEMOTHERAPY AND ADDITIONAL DRUGS

Chemotherapy is a systemic treatment approach that uses medications to target and destroy cells that divide quickly, such as cancer cells. Chemotherapy is used to treat several different medical diseases, including infections and autoimmune disorders, even though it is most commonly linked to the treatment of cancer. Chemotherapy is an effective treatment for cancer that targets cancer cells that may have migrated beyond the initial tumor since it circulates throughout the body, unlike radiation therapy or surgery.

Chemotherapy can be administered by injection, intravenous infusion, or oral medication, among other methods. The particular type, stage, and health of each patient all influence the treatment selection and combination. Frequently, the treatment plan consists of drug administration cycles interspersed with rest intervals to enable the body to recuperate from the medication's effects.

Chemotherapy frequently causes side effects, which can vary from exhaustion and immunosuppression to nausea and hair loss. The development of immunotherapy and targeted medicines, which seek to increase treatment specificity, lessen side effects, and improve overall outcomes, is a result of advancements in medical research.

CHAPTER SIX

HAVING VULVAR CANCER AND GETTING BY

CONTROLLING ADVERSE REACTIONS

It can be difficult to manage the many side effects of vulvar cancer treatment as well as the disease itself, making living with the condition a difficult journey. Managing these side effects correctly is essential to improving the general health of those with this condition. In addition to its therapies, vulvar cancer frequently causes discomfort, exhaustion, nausea, and abnormalities in the function of the bladder or intestine. A customized symptom management plan created in partnership with medical specialists can make a significant difference in reducing discomfort and enhancing day-to-day functioning.

A key component of treating vulvar cancer is pain management, for which medical professionals may suggest complementary therapies like massage or acupuncture in addition to writing prescriptions for medicine. Another common side effect, fatigue, is frequently reduced by striking a balance between rest and exercise. Gentle activity, like yoga or walking, can help you stay strong and fight off the widespread exhaustion that comes with cancer and its therapies.

SUSTAINING LIFE QUALITY

Sustaining a high standard of living is a primary objective for people managing vulvar cancer. This entails taking care of mental and psychological health in addition to treating physical problems. Creating a solid support system with friends, family, and mental health providers can help manage the psychological effects of the illness. Patients with vulvar cancer can benefit from support groups designed especially for them, which can create a sense of community by offering a forum for understanding and sharing experiences.

Many people look into complementary therapies in addition to conventional medical procedures to improve their overall quality of life. Complementary therapies, including yoga, acupuncture, or mindfulness exercises, can provide more options for treating mental and physical issues. These therapies can be incorporated into the treatment plan. These treatments are frequently selected because of their capacity to encourage calmness, lessen tension, and enhance mental wellness in general. To make sure they complement the entire treatment plan and don't conflict with medical procedures, it's imperative to go over these choices with healthcare professionals.

COMBINING COMPLEMENTARY MEDICINE

The idea of including alternative therapies in the treatment plan emphasizes the all-encompassing strategy for managing vulvar cancer. These therapies are seen to be complementary, serving different areas of well-being in conjunction with traditional treatments. The understanding that mental and emotional well-being are closely linked to physical health and that a complete approach can promote a more balanced and meaningful life both during and after treatment is the foundation for the integration of complementary treatments.

Minimizing side effects, preserving a high quality of life, and using complementary therapies are all important aspects of living with vulvar cancer. People can face the challenges of vulvar cancer with a more comprehensive and individualized approach by addressing physical symptoms, emotional well-being, and holistic techniques, ultimately improving their overall resilience and health.

CHAPTER SEVEN

INTIMACY AND SEXUALITY

HANDLING MODIFICATIONS IN SEXUAL FUNCTION

A dynamic component of human existence, sexual function can alter over time as a result of several circumstances, such as age, health, and psychological well-being. Individuals and couples must acknowledge these changes and deal with them in an honest and caring manner. For example, changes in hormone levels and physical capacities brought on by aging might affect sexual desire and performance. Sexual function can also be impacted by medical diseases like diabetes or cardiovascular problems. To comprehend the underlying causes and investigate potential treatments in such cases—whether through medical interventions, lifestyle modifications, or counseling—seeking competent medical advice is essential.

Furthermore, psychological aspects of sexual function are important. Arousal and libido can be adversely affected by stress, worry, and sadness. Addressing these issues can be made easier by having open lines of contact with medical staff or mental health specialists. A healthier sexual life can also result from partaking in activities that enhance general well-being, such as regular exercise and mindfulness exercises.

SPEAKING WITH PARTNERS

Any successful relationship starts with effective communication, which is even more important when discussing intimacy and sexuality. Partners should create a space where talking about sexual preferences, desires, and worries is greeted with compassion and understanding. Establishing a safe environment for candid communication enables people to communicate their needs and emotions without worrying about being judged. Intimacy and the emotional bond between couples can be strengthened by having open discussions about expectations, boundaries, and wishes.

Effective communication requires both partners to actively listen to each other's points of view without interrupting or assuming anything. A stronger sense of connection is fostered when people are aware of one another's wants and preferences. Recognizing that sexual tastes and desires might change over time is crucial, as is maintaining open lines of communication to make sure that each partner feels respected and appreciated in the relationship.

REGAINING CLOSENESS

Rediscovering and fostering the emotional and physical connection that may have altered or evolved is necessary to reclaim intimacy. To succeed in this process, you must be dedicated, patient, and open to trying out novel approaches to communication. It could be necessary for couples to try out other types of closeness, like non-sexual touch, verbal displays of affection, or bonding activities that are done together. Rebuilding closeness and strengthening the bond can be achieved through exploring each other's emotional landscapes and weaknesses.

Couples trying to regain intimacy may find that counseling or therapy are helpful resources. Expert advice offers a haven where spouses can discuss issues and collaborate to restore closeness. This could entail working over old grievances, developing better communication techniques, and discovering fresh approaches to making emotional and physical connections. Regaining intimacy can result in a revitalized and deeper connection that raises happiness levels in relationships overall, but it also takes work and commitment from both partners.

CHAPTER EIGHT

DIETARY ADVICE

DURING TREATMENT, NUTRITION

A healthy diet is essential for helping people receiving cancer therapy. Maintaining general health, controlling side effects, and giving the body the nutrition it needs to assist the body's coping mechanisms during therapy are the objectives. Chemotherapy and radiation therapy for cancer can frequently cause adverse symptoms like nausea, exhaustion, and changes in appetite and taste. As such, it is imperative to customize dietary recommendations to address these issues.

Sustaining a sufficient calorie intake becomes critical during cancer therapy to avoid unintentional weight loss and muscle atrophy. Foods high in vitamins and minerals and high in nutrients are recommended to boost the immune system and promote healing. Consuming protein is very important because it is essential for the immune system and tissue repair. It is advised to consume lean protein sources such as fish, poultry, tofu, and lentils.

Another important component of nutritional support for cancer patients is hydration. Consuming enough fluids aids in the management of adverse effects, such as dehydration, which some medications may make worse. Drinking water, herbal teas, and broths can help you stay hydrated generally; however, you should avoid sugar-filled drinks and too much caffeine.

PARTICULAR ATTENTION FOR PATIENTS WITH VULVAR CANCER

Patients with vulvar cancer may experience particular difficulties necessitating special dietary attention. Chemotherapy, radiation, and surgery can all have an impact on the digestive tract, which can result in problems like irregular eating patterns, trouble swallowing, and changes in bowel habits. A customized approach to diet is necessary to address these issues.

Smaller, more frequent meals might be easier to handle for patients receiving treatment for vulvar cancer than bigger ones. Smoothies, soups, and cooked veggies are examples of soft, easily digested foods that can supply vital nutrients without making you feel uncomfortable. To control bowel irregularity, one must consume enough fiber, which may be found in foods like fruits, vegetables, and whole grains.

During treatment, it's crucial to manage any possible weight fluctuations. Sustaining a healthy weight can have a good effect on general well-being and treatment results. Working together with a qualified dietitian or nutritionist can assist in developing a customized nutrition plan that takes into account the unique requirements and difficulties that individuals with vulvar cancer must overcome.

MEAL PLANS AND RECIPES

Developing wholesome and enticing dishes is essential to helping cancer patients through their treatment. Taste changes and hunger swings are common side effects, so variety and flavor become essential. The main goal of meal plans should be to provide a balance of macro and micronutrients while taking the tastes and tolerances of each individual into account.

Easy-to-digest dishes can be a fantastic choice. For instance, quinoa or brown rice combined with a protein- and vegetable-rich stir-fry makes a satisfying, well-balanced dinner. Herbs and spices can improve the flavor of food without using a lot of salt or sugar, which may need to be avoided while undergoing therapy.

A range of colorful fruits and vegetables, whole grains, lean proteins, and healthy fats should all be included in meal planning. Yogurt, berries, and leafy greens make tasty and easy-to-make smoothies that can increase nutrient consumption. In addition, energy-boosting snacks like hummus with vegetables nuts, and seeds can be consumed in between meals.

It is critical to maintain general health and well-being by customizing nutritional recommendations to the specific needs of persons undergoing cancer treatment, particularly those with vulvar cancer.

CHAPTER NINE
USEFUL ADVICE FOR EVERYDAY LIFE
HANDLING EVERYDAY DIFFICULTIES

One of the most important abilities in the complex fabric of daily life is the ability to skillfully navigate and manage the numerous problems that always arise. To begin this quest, one must first develop a robust attitude. Keeping a good attitude in the face of hardship has a big impact on one's capacity to take on obstacles head-on. It entails recognizing the obstacles, realizing that failures are a normal part of life, and actively looking for answers.

Managing your time well is another essential to overcoming everyday obstacles. Making lists of things to do, arranging tasks according to significance and urgency, and establishing reasonable objectives are all essential tools. Overwhelming jobs can appear less intimidating when broken down into smaller, more achievable steps. Creating a routine can also help to streamline daily tasks by offering stability and structure.

Having effective communication is essential for conquering obstacles. In the workplace, in interpersonal interactions, and the society, communicating wants and concerns promotes cooperation and understanding. Asking friends, family, or coworkers for support can offer insightful viewpoints and help in solving problems. Adopting a flexible mentality also promotes resilience and creativity by enabling adaptation in the face of unforeseen obstacles.

KEEPING YOUR INDEPENDENCE

Maintaining one's freedom is essential to living a happy and productive life. This calls for a multidimensional strategy that includes financial, emotional, and physical independence. The foundation of physical independence is taking responsibility for one's health. A healthy diet, regular exercise, and preventative healthcare can all enhance general well-being and help people retain their independence in day-to-day activities.

Developing self-awareness and emotional resilience is a necessary step toward emotional independence. This entails developing self-confidence, establishing sound boundaries, and identifying and controlling emotions. Developing a solid support system of friends and family in addition to taking part in happy and fulfilling activities helps improve emotional health and foster a sense of independence.

One of the main components of total freedom is financial independence. Making prudent financial decisions, sticking to a budget, and conserving money allows people to take charge of their financial future. In addition to offering stability, financial independence creates opportunities for achieving one's objectives.

MANAGING TREATMENT AND WORK

It is a delicate but necessary effort to find a balance between the demands of employment and the need for medical treatments. Having open lines of communication with employers is essential to creating a positive work atmosphere. A supportive environment can be created by outlining treatment requirements, possible accommodations, and flexible work schedules. This will assist in finding a balance between priority for your health and your commitments at work.

Managing time becomes especially important when balancing obligations to treatment and employment. Strategies such as scheduling treatment appointments during times when job stress is lower, making efficient use of breaks, and integrating self-care routines into daily schedules can aid in achieving a harmonious balance. Workplace stress can also be lessened by incorporating stress-reduction strategies like mindfulness and relaxation training.

When juggling a job and therapy, setting and upholding limits is crucial to avoiding burnout. A lasting balance is facilitated by learning to say no when it's necessary and by having reasonable expectations for both professional and health-related goals. Asking for help from friends, family, and coworkers can help you build a network of people who are sympathetic to your situation and who can assist you through this difficult balancing act.

CHAPTER TEN

RESILIENCE AND CONTINUED CARE

AFTER TREATMENT LIFE

People with cancer go through a phase known as "life after treatment," which is a major turning point in their journey. Emotions during this time can be mixed, ranging from thankfulness and relief to anxiety and uncertainty. Even though the completion of treatment is the reason for celebration, survivors frequently have to acclimate to a new normal on a physical and emotional level. Cancer has a lasting effect, and survivors may deal with issues like persistent side effects, shifting body image, and psychological fallout from the ordeal.

For numerous survivors, returning to their regular lives entails taking back facets of their lives that were momentarily halted while undergoing treatment. This can entail going back to work, getting back into social situations, and mending relationships. Healing is not just about the physical; it also involves mental and emotional health. Survivors need the safety net that comes with support from friends, family, and medical experts to get through this transitional phase and regain their footing after therapy.

FREQUENT INSPECTIONS AND SURVEILLANCE

Regular examinations and monitoring continue to be essential parts of a cancer survivor's post-treatment healthcare regimen. These follow-up meetings have several functions, such as monitoring for late-onset side effects, addressing any growing health concerns, and detecting potential cancer recurrence. The type and stage of the malignancy, the course of therapy, and personal health concerns are just a few of the variables that affect how frequently and what kind of checks are necessary.

Healthcare professionals provide comprehensive examinations, request pertinent testing, and have frank discussions regarding survivors' health and well-being during these follow-up visits. These examinations offer the chance to identify any possible problems early on, allowing for prompt intervention and increasing the likelihood of positive results. Regular monitoring also gives survivors a sense of security, enabling them to feel linked to their healthcare team and supported while they negotiate the unknowns of life beyond treatment.

PROLONGED SURVIVAL

For those who have gone beyond a certain time after finishing cancer treatment, long-term survivability is a noteworthy accomplishment. The term "long-term survivor" refers to those who have not had cancer for five years or longer, albeit the precise meaning may differ. This stage of survival entails unique issues such as maintaining health, managing medication side effects, and adopting a proactive stance towards general well-being.

Long-term cancer survivors frequently have to strike a balance between the urge to put the disease behind them and the necessity for ongoing surveillance. During this stage, lifestyle decisions including eating a balanced diet, exercising frequently, abstaining from tobacco use, and consuming moderate amounts of alcohol become critical for fostering optimum health. Survivorship care plans, which give individualized methods for managing long-term health and stress the value of constant connection with medical professionals, may also be beneficial to survivors.

Each stage of the cancer journey—life following treatment, routine check-ups, and long-term survivorship—needs to be carefully considered and supported. The shift to life after treatment is a complex process with social, emotional, and physical components. For survivors, routine examinations and monitoring provide a lifeline by enabling early detection and assistance. A celebration of tenacity and perseverance, long-term survivability encourages people to take charge of their health and cherish the time they have left before receiving cancer treatment.